Humanizing Prostate Cancer
A Physician—Patient Perspective

Humanizing Prostate Cancer
A Physician—Patient Perspective

Third Edition

Roger E. Schultz, M.D.
Physician

Alex W. Oliver
Patient

BRANDYLANE PUBLISHERS, INC.

Richmond, Virginia

❋ Brandylane Publishers, Inc.
Richmond, Virginia
www.brandylanepublishers.com

ISBN 978-1-883911-81-2

Library of Congress Control Number: 2009930021

Contents

Note from the Publisher

In addition to my professional interest in publishing the first edition of *Humanizing Prostate Cancer* (HPC), I had a keen and personal interest in the topic because my father was diagnosed with prostate cancer in the late 1960s when so much was still unknown about the disease. In spite of limited treatment options, however, he had surgery and still lived a long life. I was in my early forties when he died in 1989 at eighty-three.

When the manuscript for HPC first appeared on my desk in 1999, I knew that publishing this book would potentially help thousands of men who would be diagnosed with prostate cancer. But as a result of my father's diagnosis, I also knew I had a 50/50 chance of getting the disease, and so my interest in the book ballooned even further. I threw myself into the editing process, and learned what I could about diagnosis, treatment options and long-term prognoses. Perhaps I could take preventative measures and learn what to do if the statistical prediction of my own diagnosis turned into reality.

The painful irony is that when HPC went to a second printing in 2001, the forecast became real: I was diagnosed and had a radical prostatectomy that November. When we published the second edition two years later as a result of updated treatment options and more advanced technology, I read with different eyes. No longer was I just an editor and publisher. Now, like hundreds of thousands of other men, I was a casualty of the epidemic.

As I review this third edition of HPC in June 2009, I am still cancer free, blessed to be alive and in a position to inform men and their families that there is life after prostate cancer. I am also blessed to pass on to my two sons the importance of arming themselves with knowledge about the disease, in the event they are diagnosed themselves. But having information about the disease is only part of the ammunition to deal with a diagnosis. A man needs to communicate with his doctor, family and friends and seek their care, support and encouragement along the way. These are essential to physical and emotional healing and recovery.

Like all men who face this disease, I struggled with the impact of the doctor's words, "You have prostate cancer." Thankfully, I had this book, a well of knowledge, and my friends and family to help me through the experience, and these have made all the difference.

Robert H. Pruett
President, Brandylane Publishers, Inc.

Preface to the Third Edition

In view of recent developments in prostate cancer research and treatment, we have introduced new material into this third edition that will help men make more informed decisions about their treatment in partnership with their physicians. In part, these developments involve new drugs and refinements in procedures used for localized and advanced stages of the disease.

Research and treatment of prostate cancer are developing at a rapid rate. It is not our intention here to delve deeply into the medical and scientific aspects of new research. Instead, the purpose of this book is to present new information in a simple way that is easy to understand and that may help men and their families choose the most effective treatment in partnership with their physicians.

The material in this text is certain to change. Since the first edition was published in 2000, developments in medical technology and pharmacology have advanced how we diagnose and treat prostate cancer.

The information in this manual comes from our personal experience and training. It is a guide, but it is not a substitute for the medical opinion that you receive from your own health care provider.

Introduction

This manual is for the thousands of men who have been diagnosed with prostate cancer. Available literature about prostate cancer is often too technical and impersonal. The authors wanted to write a different kind of book to help humanize this frightening experience—a manual that is conversational in tone, easy to read, and sensitive. Their purpose is to convey important information that allows the patient to understand the disease and what can be done about it. They also wanted to talk about the mental and emotional adjustments a man must make once he's been diagnosed, because this is a vital part of healing.

This manual is more than a medical journal filled with the latest research abstracts. What makes this resource different is that it presents a dual perspective—from both a cancer survivor and the urologist who helped him. The patient, Alex Oliver's, comments provide the emotional response many men feel when faced with the diagnosis, but are often unwilling to share openly. His urologist, Roger Schultz, offers plenty of medical data and his experiences in dealing with men faced with this diagnosis. Together, they present a balanced and insightful look at a disease that has become one of the most prevalent among men.

At the least, according to the authors, this is an effort to help men, their families and friends better understand the disease and its treatment. At best, it will help calm frayed nerves and empower men to make intelligent choices about treatment and help them live full lives after treatment.

Chapter 1

Welcome to the Fraternity

You may be the one man in six who has been diagnosed this year with prostate cancer.* This is the most common solid organ cancer in men over fifty. It is not necessarily fatal. If found early, it can be treated and cured. Even when found in an advanced stage, prostate cancer can be palliated, or slowed down, with hormonal therapy. *There is something that can be done for every man who first presents with newly diagnosed prostate cancer.*

Schultz

Alex was referred to me with an elevated PSA (*prostate specific antigen*) blood test. This blood test has been used both to screen and follow the progress of men with prostate cancer. Alex had no symptoms and his prostate exam felt normal. We did a prostatic biopsy because of the blood test abnormality. Alex will tell you how he reacted.

Oliver

Sweat poured from my brow the moment he said, "You have prostate cancer." With little

*Cancer Statistics, 2008, American Cancer Society. Vol 58, No. 2, Pg. 91.

warning, this physician and this disease captivated my life. I was devastated. Why me? Why now?

Schultz

I've been giving men this news for over twenty years. There's no easy way to say it. Like most men, Alex was pretty shocked. It took time for him to get beyond the words, "prostate cancer," and to absorb any more information. Medical school teaches doctors a new language. Alex has retrained me to put this language back into common English. Most importantly he has also reminded me of the importance of humanizing the entire experience.

Oliver

Immediately my life was different. I became a recluse and my imagination went wild. For the moment, core values, logical thinking and my support group were not within reach. I was terrified.

Schultz

What Alex felt is really no different from any person who learns that he has cancer. Frankly, he was more open about his fear. Most men that I have treated initially clam up and pretend to be strong. Sometimes I meet men who insist that they don't want anyone in their family to know! These fellows would do so much better to involve their most reliable support group—their family or closest friends.

Oliver

I was so terrified, I was unsure that I could handle the situation. But I had been taught early on that it was a sign of strength to ask for help. Roger also recognized that counseling would help. Expressing my true emotions to him and letting him be part of the solution helped in making this new stranger become a trusted doctor.

Counseling pinpointed the emotional issue immediately. My fright was due to unresolved memories of my father's illness with cancer. I was six years old when he died. All I remember was his long suffering. During the 1950s, doctors didn't know much about early diagnosis and treatment. There wasn't much anyone could do, and doctors were reluctant to see him at home. Once I realized that considerable progress had been made and that his case was entirely different from mine, I began to calm down. At first, being told I had cancer meant that I was going to die. I'm glad I got help. Soon I began to think more clearly about the emotional side of the disease.

Schultz

With time, Alex became better informed about his particular case. We began to talk about the options for treatment. I recall that he would bring a list of questions at every visit. It became obvious that understanding his case helped to reduce his anxiety. In my opinion, it is vital that every man recognize that this is a common condition, that it is treatable when caught early, and that there is a fraternity of men who have been through this process and still maintain normal lives.

Oliver

Occasionally I would call Roger between office visits to ask some questions over again or to make sure I was understanding what he had told me. He always called me back promptly and never seemed bothered with my "what ifs."

> ➤ "We can do so many incredible things in medicine, but we often are far too focused on the technical issues of diagnosis and treatment. We should recognize the importance of helping patients cope, educating our patients, and involving family members."
>
> *Roger E. Schultz, M.D.*

> ➤ "The tendency to escalate a situation into its worst possible conclusion is called *awfulizing*, and it can be a key factor in tipping the balance toward illness or health." (Joan Borysenko in *Minding the Body/Mending the Mind*)
>
> ➤ Remember, "Make the mind command the body. . . Fear kills more people than death." (General Patton)

Schultz

Fear and panic are not constructive emotions. You get better results when you keep your head on straight.

Oliver

In the ensuing weeks that led to surgery, I delved deeply into the physical, mental and emotional aspects of the disease. Soon I became comfortable with what I had to do and confident in my *urologist*. By surgery day, I was ready. In fact, the surgery went beautifully and very much as he had described to me.

> ➤ "Generally, bad news makes the best headlines,"
> says Chris Matthews in *Hardball.* The good news is
> that thousands of men who have been diagnosed
> with the disease are living normal lives.
>
> *Alex W. Oliver*

Schultz

We chose surgery for Alex based on his young age, excellent health and clinical circumstances. I believe that Alex did well because he was very prepared and very comfortable with his decision. He was soon back to a normal routine as I had anticipated.

Oliver

In the time since my surgery, I have spoken with numerous men who have been diagnosed with prostate cancer. While each individual has different concerns, there is one similar response—fear!

Schultz

We are convinced that the fear factor can be minimized by the patient and doctor forming a good working relationship. In the best of circumstances, the physician is unhurried and empathetic. It may take several visits to develop a comfort level that permits truly meaningful communication. If the physician can provide his patient with information about the therapy and its risks, the patient will be better prepared to deal with any potential problems or unforeseen circumstances. Also, if a patient is armed with information about the potential risks of therapy, he will be better prepared to deal with any problems that arise following therapy.

_____ *Oliver*

The relationship with your doctor can be established by being yourself. I liked knowing that he always had good eye contact with me. I was a real person and not just one more name in his patient charts.

> O.K. So now you know you have prostate cancer. At least you know. Just think of the number of men who have it and don't yet know.

> Try not to compare your case, treatment, and/or recovery with anyone else. Each man's story is different.

Alex W. Oliver

Chapter 2

Don't Believe Everything You Hear

Schultz

Alex was troubled by all the hearsay about prostate cancer. Like other men, he couldn't get a handle on what was fact and what was fiction.

Oliver

Once I began to sort the facts and understand my specific case, I began to relax. Contrary to the myth, considerable progress has been made in the detection and treatment of prostate cancer. Many of us who have joined the fraternity are now able to benefit from the more recent research and developments in treatment.

Schultz

First, let's begin by identifying the location of the prostate.

The prostate sits beneath the bladder and surrounds the urethra.

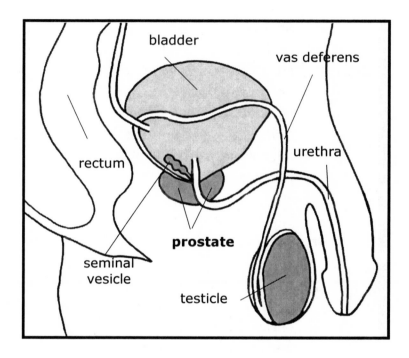

We feel that it is important to point out some of the ideas about this disease that are false.

Exploring the Myths and Realities

The prostate's job is to help with sex.

> After puberty, the prostate makes semen. After age fifty, it makes trouble! It is the most common organ to develop cancer in men over fifty. The prostate has nothing to do with sex drive, erections, and orgasm. The nerves and blood vessels that go to the penis pass on either side of the prostate. Injury to these structures, but not the prostate itself, can lead to problems with erections.

There must be something in the air or water. More men are getting the disease.

> We are finding more cases of prostate cancer because of the PSA (Prostate Specific Antigen) test and a greater awareness about the disease. Fatty foods may be related, but not the air or water. You are at greater risk of developing prostate cancer if you are older, African-American, or have a father or brother with the same disease.

This is an old man's disease, so I can ignore it until I retire.

Not true! With the arrival of the PSA blood test, doctors have identified men in their forties and fifties who have normal prostate examinations and no symptoms. The biopsies of their prostates often show higher grades of cancer, sometimes lots of it, too.

Get a PSA test, but forget the rectal exam!

These tests complement one another, so both should be done. About 25% of men with prostate cancer have a normal PSA. The cancer may show up as a nodule (hard spot) felt by examination. So don't talk your doctor out of the *digital rectal exam.*

Prostate cancer is slow growing and you'll outlive it,
so why bother looking for it.

This might be true for a very old man with a tiny area of prostate cancer found on a biopsy. On the other hand, it might be risky for a healthy fifty-year-old to ignore his diagnosis and take the chance that the tumor will never affect him. Why? Because the cancer inevitably grows. Once the cancer spreads, there is no treatment that will cure or eliminate the cancer. Advanced disease can be painful and costly. In later chapters we will review how the *grade* and the *volume* of cancer affect prognosis.

Life is never the same after treatment. Your sex life ends and you leak urine constantly.

If we treat a man whose cancer is confined to the prostate, he will likely return to a normal working life. Treatment for advanced stages will generally control the tumor and either improve or delay the appearance of symptoms such as bone pain, urinary bleeding or urinary obstruction.

Impotence (inability to get good erections) may occur with treatment. The newer techniques (e.g., nerve sparing surgery, conformal radiation, and brachytherapy) can lessen the likelihood of impotence. There are many different ways to treat men with erectile dysfunction, so don't write off your sex life!

Urinary incontinence (leakage) rarely occurs with radiation, but might occur after surgery. Some men will have stress incontinence— leakage that occurs with coughing or swinging a golf club. This often improves with time, and it can be treated if it persists. Your age, body build, and general health influence this potential problem, so you should discuss this issue with your urologist.

I have to have my treatment at a cancer institute.

If your Ford breaks down, do you take it to Detroit for repairs? Having a choice of treatments is better than no choice at all, but it does create confusion and anxiety. I often advise patients to seek a second or third opinion from other doctors, including those at major medical centers. Once you decide on treatment, then you must choose the treating doctor. This depends on your confidence in your physician. Does he have credentials? Is he well regarded by his medical peers? Does he take time to explain? Does he listen to you? A busy community *urologist* or *radiation oncologist* may provide care that is as good as the cancer centers. You will need someone to call if you have any problems related to your treatment. And you will need follow-up to be sure that you remain free of cancer. This is a lot more easily done if you develop a relationship with a doctor near your home and hospital.

We haven't made much progress in the diagnosis or treatment of this disease.

Not so! I can show you major developments in both diagnosis and treatment.

In the area of diagnosis, the PSA blood test has allowed earlier detection. Ultrasound allows us to see deep inside the prostate gland.

Biopsy instruments are smaller, faster, and less painful.

In the treatment arena, surgery is more routine than ever. Because of newer techniques, complications, particularly urinary incontinence and erectile dysfunction, are much less common. Conformal *external beam irradiation* allows the treating doctor to wrap the radiation around the prostate, minimizing risk to the nearby organs like the bladder and rectum. *Brachytherapy*, the placement of radioactive seeds in the prostate, has become attractive due to improved imaging that allows very accurate distribution of seeds. Chemotherapy has shown improved response rates even in cases that would not respond to other treatments.

Unique medical delivery systems, such as *Vantas*, are designed to treat symptoms of advanced prostate cancer while providing the convenience of a once a year dose.

Genetic research is the hot subject today. We may soon be able to analyze genes and their protein by-products to predict future risk and stage of this disease. Our hope is that we will develop targeted therapies that correct or delete "bad genes" or the proteins produced by these genes that allow cancers to grow.

Chapter 3

A New Chapter in Your Life

Oliver

Please note that we call this "A New Chapter in Your Life" not "The Last Word." What we offer in this chapter are basic facts, many of which may be new to you. Understanding the diagnosis will help you to determine the course of treatment. We believe having a basic understanding will also help quiet the alarm bell.

Understanding the Diagnosis

Schultz

A tumor is a growth that occurs in a body organ that may or may not be life threatening. Speaking very generally, a benign tumor usually remains confined to the same organ from which it began. A malignant tumor is one that can grow out of control and spread to other organs. A malignant tumor is called a cancer. When cancer spreads to other organs, it can interfere with the function of those organs. It can weaken the body's immune system, that is, the ability to fight off even simple infections. The cancer saps the nutrition from healthy cells and can cause weight loss and weakness. People die from cancer for many reasons, but the most common ones are severe infections and the failure of multiple organs.

Remember that early prostate cancer may cause no symptoms. We have already discussed the importance of an annual *digital rectal examination* and *PSA blood test* for those men who wish to screen for prostate cancer. The PSA blood test can be falsely elevated by benign prostatic enlargement or prostatitis (inflammation). Passing instruments or catheters into the bladder may elevate it. It is not elevated by simple rectal examination of the prostate. If there is any question regarding the validity of the PSA result, I would repeat it. Bacterial prostatitis (genital pain, tender prostate) can generally be treated with an antibiotic such as *Levaquin*. Non-bacterial prostatitis often responds to tub soaks, anti-inflammatory medicine and reduced physical activity. I often wait six weeks following treatment for prostatitis to see whether the PSA falls to normal. If the digital rectal examination or the PSA remains abnormal, we would advise a prostate biopsy under ultrasound guidance. This is an office-based test that takes just fifteen minutes. We pass an ultrasound probe about two inches in the rectum and use it to guide a biopsy device to several areas of the prostate. The instrument has a small needle and takes samples quickly. Multiple biopsies (ten or more cores) are taken to see if cancer is present and to estimate its extent in the prostate (volume of disease). There is some discomfort and often a desire to urinate. I rarely use sedatives for this procedure, but I do inject a numbing drug into the nerves on either side of the prostate.

> ➤ You don't have to play Tarzan when going through therapy. Let your body tell you what you can do. Learn to relax and work on total self-healing.
>
> *Alex W. Oliver*

Oliver

I took an antibiotic for a few days to prevent a bacterial infection that could occur after passing a biopsy needle through the rectal wall. There was no pain resulting from my test. I didn't see any blood in my urine, but I know of several friends who noticed blood in the urine for a few days. I was tired but that was caused by my anxiety.

> ➤ Part of the fraternity initiation is experiencing "data shock" (*So much new information to understand so quickly*). Let your physician help you through the crisis. He is on your side and is your best resource. Ask questions.
>
> *Alex W. Oliver*

Schultz

Cancer is usually diagnosed by a *pathologist*, a physician skilled at recognizing cancer when the specimens are viewed under a microscope. He will assign a *grade* to the cancer. This is an attempt to judge how aggressive the cancer may behave. The grade is based on the appearance of the cells and their relationship to other cells.

One of the most popular grading systems was described by *Gleason*. He defines five microscopic patterns of prostate cancer and gives each pattern a number from one (least aggressive) to five (most aggressive). He then adds the two most common patterns seen under the microscope, giving him the *Gleason score*. A low Gleason score (e.g., 3+2=5) generally has a better prognosis than a high Gleason score (e.g., 4+5=9). Like pieces of a puzzle, the combination of PSA level, Gleason score, and tumor volume tell us about tumor behavior.

Staging the Disease

We discover prostate cancer at different stages. The *stage* refers to the location of the cancer relative to the rest of the body. Is the cancer well within the borders of the prostate? Has it broken through the prostate capsule into the fatty tissue around the prostate? Has it spread to other organs (e.g., the bones or the lungs)?

There are two staging systems that are popular among physicians. The first is the *Whitmore-Jewett system* of four stages (A, B, C & D). The other is the *TNM system* which is more universally known and shown in Table 1. The "T" refers to tumor size. The "N" refers to the lymph node status. The "M" refers to the presence of metastases (cancer spread).

Using the TNM system, we categorize a man with cancer found only by way of elevated PSA as a stage T1. If there is a nodule, it is a T2. A larger cancer has a higher T number. With regard to spread to lymph nodes and other organs, we will often order a CAT scan of the pelvis, a bone scan, a chest X-ray, and blood tests that check your blood count or liver function. Recent clinical research has shown that many of these tests are not needed if the Gleason score is less than 6 and the PSA is less than 10 ng/ml. In this instance, the likelihood of finding cancer beyond the prostate is so low

TABLE 1: TNM System for Staging Prostate Cancer

T ➤ **Primary Tumor**

TX ➤ Primary tumor cannot be assessed.

T1 ➤ Cannot feel tumor or see it using imaging (x-ray or ultrasound). Cancer found in specimen after a transurethral resection of prostate. Cancer found on a biopsy done only because of an elevated PSA test.

T2 ➤ Tumor is confined to the prostate.

T3 ➤ Tumor breaks through the capsule of the prostate or invades the seminal vesicles.

T4 ➤ Tumor invades structures other than the seminal vesicles.

N ➤ **Regional Lymph Nodes**

NX ➤ Regional lymph nodes cannot be assessed.

N0 ➤ Regional lymph nodes do not show cancer present.

N1 ➤ Regional lymph nodes contain cancer.

M ➤ **Distant metastasis (cancer spread)**

MX ➤ Distant metastases cannot be assessed.

M0 ➤ No distant metastases seen.

M1 ➤ Distant metastases are present.

that these tests may be a waste of time and money. A nuclear scan, called Prostascint, has also been developed to look for the spread of prostate cancer. It has not been universally accepted for staging. It can be useful for finding recurrent cancer after treatment.

Much like the chapter on therapy, you can find a multitude of blood and imaging studies that could be done, but someone educated in the treatment of this disease needs to help you choose those tests that assist decision-making and minimize anxiety.

Chapter 4

Choices and Challenges

Oliver

My first reaction to the diagnosis was to do something quickly. In most cases you will have time to determine what is best for you. Don't panic. Get the facts. There may be several treatment options. I had three choices. My wife and I agreed that surgery was my best option. The doctor agreed. The three of us were partners in making the medical decision.

My friends tell me I was totally absorbed in this crisis and they didn't know how to help. I didn't know any man who had survived prostate cancer. More discussion would have helped.

Schultz

How do you pick a plan for the treatment of prostate cancer? In the medical community you could speak to your family doctor, urologist, or radiation oncologist. You could do research in the medical library, only to be frustrated by medical technotalk. Others surf the Web and find reams of data. Or you could contact sources who provide integrative medicine. Unfortunately, there are very few clinical trials that prove that alternative approaches alone will cure prostate cancer. On the other hand, there is data to suggest that proper exercise, nutrition, and stress reduction will strengthen the body and boost its immune system.

First and foremost, I suggest that you find a physician whom you trust and who is an expert in this disease. Seek additional opinions if you feel so inclined. Talk to friends or survivors within support groups (like Us Too or Man to Man. See below), but recognize that their circumstances are not always comparable to your own. Get your loved ones involved. If you are supported, if you collect information that can be sorted and interpreted, if you trust your advisors, then you will be able to take charge, make a decision, and promote your own healing. Let's explore each option and look at some examples.

Prostate Cancer Support Groups

Call to find out local chapter information.

Man to Man

Supported by the American Cancer Society

800-ACS-2345 • www.cancer.org

Us Too International

800-808-7866 • www.ustoo.org

Prostate Cancer Foundation

800-757-2873 • www.prostatecancerfoundation.org

> There is no best approach for all cancers. The first thing I tell patients is that they have to decide whether they will treat the disease or not. If they choose treatment, then they can select from a menu of options. The decision to treat will depend upon multiple issues: the age and general mental, emotional and physical health of the patient, the grade/stage of disease, the PSA level, and the expectations and fears of the individual.
>
> *Roger E. Schultz, M.D.*

Active Surveillance

Schultz

No treatment is provided unless the cancer shows increased activity. Typically the tumor is very small. The pathologist has given it a low Gleason score. Your PSA may be normal or only minimally elevated. In this case, we would keep an eye on the PSA and clinical signs and symptoms. Should there be a dramatic change in either, we could start treatment. Sometimes we will do a second prostate biopsy one or two years after the original biopsy, which can help in the decision process. If the second biopsy is negative, we would not treat. If there is much more cancer seen, we would advise active treatment.

Example: A seventy-two year old man has a *transurethral resection of the prostate* (*TURP*, "ream-job") to help him urinate more easily. Although his PSA and prostate exam are normal, the tissue removed shows a tiny spot of cancer in less than 1% of the specimen (Gleason score = 5). He chooses no treatment. Over time there is no change in the PSA or prostate exam. He continues to urinate easily and has no problems related to his prostate.

> ➤ The benefit of observation only is clearly the lack of any of the side effects or the expense of treatment. The disadvantage is the remote possibility of cancer progressing and spreading to other areas of the body.
>
> *Roger E. Schultz*

External Beam Irradiation

Schultz

If the prostate tumor is T3 or less and there is no spread of disease, you may benefit from this form of therapy. Many good studies indicate that the use of hormonal shots given in and around the time of the radiation may shrink the prostate and improve the response to the radiation, particulary in men with high grades of cancer or higher PSA values. The radiation oncologist would decide the proper dosing of radiation. You would be scheduled to come back daily for a brief exposure to radiation aimed at the prostate. The newest technique of conformal therapy allows them to wrap the radiation around the prostate in a way that minimizes radiation scatter to the nearby bladder or rectum. The radiation must be given in small amounts over about an eight week period. It destroys the tumor while leaving the prostate in place. The results are judged by the prostate exam (it often feels flat after treatment) and the PSA level. The PSA "nadir" (the lowest level to which the PSA should decrease) is debatable. Ideally it should fall to less than 0.5 ng/ml. Regardless of the absolute value, all agree that the PSA should not rise from its lower baseline over several consecutive visits. A PSA that continually rises off its new baseline suggests that the cancer is still active.

Example: A seventy-two year old man has a hard area involving the entire right side of the prostate. The PSA is 8ng/ml. Biopsy confirms a cancer with a Gleason score = 6. He has coronary artery disease and diabetes that is controlled with insulin.

In this example, surgery may not be ideal. First of all, his heart disease and diabetes increase the risk of surgical complications (heart attack, infection). Second, if the tumor is large and may extend beyond the confines of the prostate he may need additional therapy, possibly radiation! So it may be wiser to direct this man to radiation first.

Brachytherapy

Schultz

Brachytherapy or interstitial irradiation is the placement of radioactive "seeds" directly in the prostate gland. The seeds emit radiation that kills prostate cancer cells, then they "burn out." Over time the seeds lose their radioactivity and remain in the prostate gland forever.

During the past several years there has been a surge in brachytherapy because of improved techniques to map the prostate using computers and because of improved delivery systems using ultrasound. Brachytherapy is a cooperative effort between the urologist and the radiation oncologist. We first measure the prostate volume by placing an ultrasound probe in the rectum. Multiple images are taken and a computer helps to determine the total volume. These measurements help us decide how many seeds may be needed to treat the entire gland. We order the seeds and schedule the treatment itself. On the day of treatment you are taken to the operating room, given an anesthetic and placed in stirrups. A grid is placed up against the perineum (area between the scrotal sac and the rectum). We put the ultrasound probe in the rectum to identify the prostate and guide the process. Needles are placed through the holes in the grid and seeds are then passed down the center of these needles into the prostate gland. We remove the needles leaving the seeds behind. You go home the same day. Some doctors combine external beam irradiation and brachytherapy for higher grade (more aggressive) cancer.

Example: A sixty-seven-year-old healthy man has a small prostate with a nodule. Biopsy confirms a Gleason score = 5 in the nodule only. This patient wants to be cured, and he wants a minimally invasive approach to therapy. Although he could choose external beam radiation or surgery, he opts instead for brachytherapy. Many studies show that this out-patient treatment is as good as surgery or external beam radiation.

The surgical removal of prostate cancer is called a *radical prostatectomy*. The term *radical* refers to the complete removal of the entire prostate and *seminal vesicles*. People ask why we can't remove the cancerous area and leave the normal prostate gland alone. This is because prostate cancer is often found or may develop in multiple areas within the gland. It is also technically harder to cut out a segment of this single, centrally placed organ.

The nerves that go to the penis to provide an erection sit alongside the prostate. When possible, the surgeon will try to protect these nerves as he removes the prostate. When the prostate has been removed, the surgeon must sew the bladder to the urethral stump. A urethral catheter is left in place from 1-3 weeks until the connection between the bladder and urethra has a watertight seal. The operation takes about two to four hours. The hospital stay is about one to three days.

Some surgeons offer laparoscopic prostatectomy as a less invasive means of removing the prostate. The use of robotic arms placed through the laparoscopic ports allows the surgeon to perform a much more precise repair using magnification. When done very well there is less post-operative pain, earlier removal of the urethral catheter, and often earlier return of urinary continence. Laparoscopic surgery, with or without the robot, does not necessarily cure the cancer any better than open surgery. This equipment is very expensive and is not available at most hospitals at this time.

Why would you choose surgery instead of radiation? Surgery is faster (two to four hours vs. eight weeks for external beam irradiation). Surgery is the only way to actually hand examine and learn more about the patient's prognosis. Some argue that surgery provides a better cure rate, particularly if the tumor appears aggressive (high Gleason score). Nerve sparing surgery may permit a greater likelihood of erections after treatment. Finally, if cancer shows up again in the pelvis, you can undergo radiation to this area. The reverse is not as easy. If you have recurrent cancer after radiation treatment, it is not possible to undergo more pelvic irradiation, and surgery on tissues that have received radiation is very difficult.

Example: A fifty-year-old athletic man is sent to us following annual physical because his PSA = 5.0 ng/ml. He has no symptoms and his prostate feels normal.

Biopsy confirms a Gleason score 7 prostate cancer in three of twelve cores sent. He is potent and wants to remain so! He would have a high likelihood of cure with few complications if he chose surgery.

30

Cryoablative Surgery

This out-patient procedure involves regional or general anesthesia. The surgeon places multiple needles through the perineum (area between the scrotum and anus) into the prostate. These probes are frozen to about -40 degrees, thawed, frozen again, then thawed and removed. The ice ball created will kill the prostate tissue, including the cancer. To monitor the process, the doctor places an ultrasound guide in the rectum. Newer and smaller probes have enabled more precise localization and reduced likelihood of injury to the rectum or urinary sphincter. The nerves outside the prostatic capsule are usually frozen, so erectile impotence is very likely to occur. I prefer this therapy for men with poor sexual function.

It is possible to freeze a very small area of the prostate that may be the only site of cancer. This so-called "focal cryotherapy" has been marketed by some centers as the "male lumpectomy" (the equivalent of a breast lump removal instead of a complete mastectomy in a female). It is appealing because it will spare the nerves on the untreated side of the prostate and possibly preserve erectile potency. Critics of focal cryotherapy argue that it may under-treat this often multifocal cancer.

High Intensity Focused Ultrasound

High Intensity Focused Ultrasound (HIFU) is a newer, but not necessarily better, treatment of early prostate cancer. This out-patient procedure requires some anesthesia. A special ultrasound probe is placed in the rectum and the focused ultrasound energy causes thermal injury in small, overlapping areas of the prostate. It is minimally invasive and involves no radiation. As of this edition, HIFU is not yet FDA approved in the US. More data must be examined to see if HIFU will be as effective as other treatments.

Hormonal deprivation

Schultz
_____

Prostate cancer is sensitive to the effects of testosterone, a hormone produced mostly by the testicles and a little by the adrenal glands. We can slow down the activity of prostate cancer by removing the testicles (*orchiectomies*). This is done as an outpatient and takes about thirty minutes. Newer medications called LHRH agonists (*Vantas, Zoladex, Lupron, Eligard, Trelstar*) provide an alternative to the removal of the testicles. These drugs reduce levels of male hormone. Zoladex, Lupron, Eligard and Trelstar are shots that are given in the office every one to six months depending upon the preparation. They are given for the lifetime of the patient. One unique product, *Vantas*, represents a small implant of medicine housed in a one-inch tubular polymer, the same type of material used in contact lenses. The urologist places the implant under the skin of the upper arm. The drug is slowly released over twelve months, then the implant is removed and may be replaced. Many men choose *Vantas* for the convenience of once a year dosing.

All drugs that lower testosterone can cause hot flashes, erectile dysfunction and bone loss.

Newer data shows that LHRH agonists also lead to higher cholesterol levels and insulin resistance. I advise men who use any of these drugs to take calcium and Vitamin D and to exercise regularly to protect their bones from injury.

Some, but not all, doctors believe that the small amount of testosterone generated by the adrenal gland should also be eliminated to maximize survival. This can be done using oral drugs called *antiandrogens* (Eulexin, Casodex, Nilandron). The combination of an LHRH agonist and an antiandrogen is referred to as *complete androgen blockade*. There is a small survival advantage for some men who choose complete androgen blockade, but the addition of an anti-androgen can be prohibitively expensive and is not currently covered by Medicare.

Hormonal deprivation alone is not typically offered to a man with a potentially curable cancer. Although the cancer may shrink away initially, it will eventually become resistant to the effects of orchiectomies or LHRH shots. Unresponsive cells start to grow and can cause urinary symptoms or spread farther.

Example: A sixty-five-year-old man has some trouble voiding. His prostate is not large, but it is uniformly rock hard. His PSA is 45 ng/ml! Biopsy confirms a Gleason score 9 cancer in nine of ten cores sent. A bone scan shows "hot spots" (*metastases*) in numerous areas in his ribs and pelvic bones.

Neither prostatectomy, radiation, cryotherapy or HIFU will cure him. Hormonal deprivation gives a high likelihood of controlling the growth of his cancer for several months or possibly several years. He will likely experience a recurrence (more cancer shows up again later).

Chemotherapy

Schultz

Chemotherapy is not a primary treatment for most prostate cancers. It is generally reserved for cases in which hormonal deprivation has failed (called Hormonally Refractory Prostate Cancer). Available chemotherapy may slow tumor growth and control pain.

The prognosis for cancers that do not respond to chemotherapy is poor.

Some of the drugs used alone, or in combination, include Prednisone, Mitoxantrone, Docetaxel, Estramustine, and Satraplatin. Oncologists are now studying targeted therapies that interfere with angiogenesis (growth of tumor blood vessels) and tumor growth factors. Immunotherapy (the use of specific vaccines, antibodies, and immunostimulants) is also an area of intense research at this time.

Although intended for advanced disease, many investigators believe that we will eventually adopt a multimodal approach (use of chemotherapy/ immunotherapy with surgery or radiation) for earlier stage disease.

Zolendronic acid (Zometa) has been approved for patients who have prostate cancer in the bones (metastatic disease). This intravenous drug is not chemotherapy. It is given monthly in the doctor's office to reduce the complications of bone fracture, the need for radiation to treat bone pain, and the need for bone surgery to an already weakened bone.

_____ *Oliver*

In my case, the doctor suggested several choices for therapy. What is most important is that we made the final decision for surgery together.

What Would You Do, Doc?

Tough question. First, you and your medical advisors must be confident that the tumor is a risk to your health; otherwise you may suffer the side effects of treatment for little gain. Older men, in particular, may have competing medical problems that could take them to heaven long before the prostate cancer ever hurts them. So consider monitoring the cancer and treating only if there is obvious progression.

Riskier cancers demonstrate the following features: steadily rising PSA values, or worse, a doubling of PSA values, high Gleason score (7-10), large cancer size, multifocality (cancer seen in many biopsy cores), and metastases (spread beyond the prostate). Younger men with cancer may wish to undergo treatment because they have a long time horizon during which time the cancer can grow and potentially spread.

As for the best treatment for early (localized) disease, the answer is not clear. There are very few head-to-head studies that compare men who had a prostatectomy to others who had external beam radiation, seed implants, or cryotherapy. The results of each treatment type are available, and they compare well to each other in terms of cancer control. In my mind, the decision is not about which cures better, but rather how you feel about the type of treatment and its side effects. You should also consider your bail out plan if the primary treatment fails to fully cure the cancer.

Chapter 5

We Thought You'd Never Ask!

If you don't learn anything else from our manual, please remember to ask your doctor as many questions as you need answers. We've even done some thinking for you by giving you eighteen questions and answers. If there are others, write them down and ask them during your next visit.

Schultz

Your doctor sees a great number of patients on a regular basis. Don't expect him to anticipate all of your questions. It is up to you to get the facts you need in making the best decision. Remember, the only dumb questions are the ones you didn't ask!

Eighteen Questions for Your Physician

1. What is the normal range for the PSA (prostate specific antigen) blood test?

The value for PSA increases with age. There are several different methods of measuring PSA, so you must ask your doctor about his lab's reference ranges. The "normal" value of the PSA varies with age. PSA tends to go higher as you get older.

A PSA = 4.0 may be abnormally high for a forty year old, but well within the normal range for a seventy year old. The rate of change of PSA from test to test is also important. A rapidly rising PSA between doctor visits can also indicate a possible cancer. If your PSA is borderline and/or slowly rising, we may order a *Percent Free-PSA* blood test. This measures how much PSA is free versus how much is bound to other blood proteins. If your Percent Free–PSA is low (low is abnormal), you may need a prostate biopsy.

2. How do I know whether my doctor is qualified to advise or treat me?

You should certainly lean on your family physician for initial guidance. He will likely steer you to a urologist, a radiation oncologist, or both. Look for board certification, a qualification that tells you that the doctor has passed some difficult exams given by his peers. Ask what his/her experience has been treating prostate cancer. Ask if there is a similar patient in his practice who would be willing to speak to you about his experience.

➢ Don't expect your doctor to speak in absolute terms. "Always" and "never" are not in his vocabulary.

Alex W. Oliver

3. Who else could I contact for information?

There are Prostate Cancer Support groups (Us Too, Man to Man and others) in most areas with larger populations. Some other suggestions include the Prostate Cancer Network of the American Foundation for Urologic Diseases (800-828-7866), The National Cancer Institute (800-4-CANCER) and The American Cancer Society (800-ACS-2345), and Cancer Care (800-813-4673).

4. How quickly must I act?

This depends on your PSA level, your biopsy report, your health, and your anxiety level. In cases of early detection, there is very limited risk in waiting several weeks to gather information. You should be able to get it all together within a few weeks. More advanced cases may need more urgent treatment.

5. What happens if I don't do anything?

Again, this depends on the status of your disease (PSA level, Gleason score, cancer volume). If you have early disease and no symptoms, you might not have any problems for months or even years. In most instances, prostate cancer grows slowly, but it invariably grows! Once the disease is more advanced, it can cause a variety of symptoms: urinary (weak stream, urgent need to void, bloody urine), bone pain, obstructed kidneys, weight loss, and weakness.

6. How much should I tell my family, friends, and co workers?

In our opinion, you should involve your closest family members or friends in the decision process. Who else cares more for you? There is no shame in telling your friends or work mates who ask about your condition. You may prompt them to get a check-up also!

7. Can I hurt myself or my partner by having sex?

Prostate cancer is not contagious! Sexual intimacy of any kind will not make your cancer worse, nor will it cause any harm to your partner.

8. Does insurance pay for the tests and the treatment for prostate cancer?

Your medical insurance will pay unless your doctor orders unusual or uncommon tests or treatments. If you are concerned, call your insurance carrier before you proceed.

9. Doesn't radical prostatectomy cause incontinence and impotence?

You need a seasoned surgeon to get good results. Continual urinary leakage should be very rare. Some men will have stress incontinence, a little drip when they are physically active. Obese men have a greater risk of urinary leakage after surgery.

The nerve sparing prostatectomy really does work. Erectile function can take up to a year or more to fully return. Best results are in younger, very potent men. Men over the age of seventy may not retain the quality of erections they had earlier.

10. Should I have an open prostatectomy or a laparoscopic, robotic prostatectomy?

The use of a laparoscope allows the surgeon to make smaller skin incisions and work with a magnified field of view. Using a robot, the bladder neck can be sewn to the urethra with a nice water-tight suture-line. Patients go home and get rid of their urinary catheters sooner than they typically do with open surgery. Overall recovery is faster.

There is no evidence that robotic assisted surgery provides any better cure or fewer long term complications than open surgery. Some critics of the robotic procedure argue that there may be a higher rate of positive margins (cancer left behind) because the operating surgeon sees, but cannot feel, what he is cutting. This debate will sort out more fully as we collect more outcome data.

11. What are the side effects of radiation?

The bladder and rectum can be affected by radiation "scatter." This translates into urinary urgency/frequency and rectal discomfort/ diarrhea. These symptoms can be treated and they usually disappear once the radiation treatment has been completed. Some men develop troublesome, long term rectal or bladder bleeding.

12. Why doesn't everyone select brachytherapy or cryoablation or HIFU if it they are done as an outpatient procedure?

If you wish to avoid or cannot undergo surgery, this is a viable alternative. These procedures cannot be easily done in very large prostates because we will be unable to treat the entire gland, especially that portion that projects above the pubic bone. In some cases, the gland can be shrunk using LHRH drugs and will become small enough for these approaches. Patients who have had previous prostate surgery are also poor candidates for brachytherapy because it is difficult to place the seeds. The cryotherapy probes have been improved, but some doctors are waiting for more long term data that proves that it is as effective as radiation or surgery. Cryotherapy has a high rate of erectile dysfunction. HIFU is not FDA approved in the US.

13. What do I do if surgery fails to control the cancer?
If radiation fails?

Some men will benefit from external beam radiation after surgery if the pathologist tells us that the cancer has spread outside the prostate capsule or into the seminal vesicles. If the cancer shows up in the pelvis years after surgery (slowly rising PSA seen, or a rectal mass evident), you might also need external beam irradiation. If the cancer returns in a more distant location—*metastatic disease*—you will need hormonal treatment.

If there is a pelvic recurrence after radiation of any kind, you have a bigger problem. You cannot receive additional radiation. "Salvage prostatectomy" can be done, but the surgery of irradiated tissue is difficult. Complications of impotence and incontinence are much higher after salvage surgery. Cryotherapy or HIFU is an option, but there is not much data to wholeheartedly advise it. Hormonal treatment is often advised as *palliation*—that is, an effort to control the tumor and the symptoms it may produce.

14. Which is better for palliation of advanced disease—removal of testicles (orchiectomies) or use of medication (LHRH)?

Neither is better. Both accomplish the same thing by lowering male hormone levels. There is no benefit to doing both orchiectomies and LHRH agonists. The choice is strictly a personal one. Removal of the testicles takes thirty minutes in the operating room. It is a one-time treatment, and it is permanent. The LHRH shots must be given every several months. The *Vantas* implant lasts an entire year and must be replaced. LHRH agonists are expensive but generally covered by insurance.

15. What is pulse or intermittent therapy using LHRH agonists?

The current standard of care is the continuous use of LHRH agonists for the lifetime of the patient. Some doctors are administering the drug only if and when there are changes in the PSA, exam, or symptoms. This would lessen the cost and side effects of these drugs.

16. What can I do to prevent prostate cancer?

Stay on a diet that is low in animal fat. Based on some encouraging but limited data, some patients may wish to use selenium, Vitamins D & E, soy and lycopene. Several national studies are underway to provide more conclusive evidence to support their use. Drugs used to treat benign prostate enlargement (Proscar, Avodart) may have a protective role, but there is not yet an approved indication for their use in the prevention of this disease.

17. If I have had prostatitis, am I at increased risk for prostate cancer?

Maybe. What is clear is that prostatitis can cause an elevation of your PSA test. Several weeks after treatment for prostatitis (e.g., using an antibiotic like *Levaquin,* tub soaks, reduced physical/sexual activity), the PSA usually returns to a normal value. If it does not normalize, a biopsy may be necessary.

18. I get mailings about drugs that improve prostate health. Most of these drugs are non-prescription. Do they work?

In my opinion, the unsolicited mailings are simply ads. Most doctors have been taught to use medication that has clear benefits when compared to a placebo (a blank pill containing no medicine). There is little or no data to suggest that a non-prescription drug will cure prostate cancer any better than a placebo.

Chapter 6

Getting It Together

Schultz

The medical profession has made significant advances in the treatment of prostate cancer. One of the most important findings is that men who are prepared mentally, physically, and spiritually do much better with treatment and recovery. Alex is a good example of a young man who worked through the fright and anger stages and did well with treatment.

Oliver

Take a quick look at the front cover. What does the yellow square with the red dot mean to you? Responses will vary, but there is a 99.5% chance that your answer had something to do with the red dot.

Is there a lesson to this exercise? You bet! Think of the square as your total life. Don't allow the red dot to overshadow the yellow surface.

To be more specific, don't let prostate cancer become your life. Easy to say? Harder to do? Yes! Take it from one whose life became a red square for a while. And, boy, was it unnecessary!

So take a few tips from one who learned the hard way.

Avoid fantasizing about what could happen.

Ask your doctor specific questions that can reduce the fear. Write down the answers. Every time you find yourself slipping into the fear zone, read the "awfulizing" quote on page 5.

Learn what you must let go and what you can control.

This was hard for me, a professional control freak. It didn't take long to find out that the doctor, the quarterback, was in charge of much of my life. What helped me was understanding what I could control: my physical and spiritual well-being; my understanding of the disease and my particular case; and my handling of my work and social schedule to meet the requirements of appointments and testing schedule. In short, I could be in control of life up to a point. But it was fine with me for Roger to be my partner in making medical decisions. I had confidence in him.

Have confidence in your doctor.

Although I did not know Roger Schultz, I knew his reputation in the medical community and knew other men he had treated. Roger told me that surgery had been fine-tuned and that I would very likely do well. He was right.

I had surgery on a Thursday morning. By Friday afternoon I was up and doing some walking. I ate well and slept comfortably. By Sunday afternoon I was home. Monday I sat at a card table and did a limited amount of work. I experienced little pain and noted an increase in strength every day. Two weeks later the catheter was removed. No big deal. No pain.

Today I would have chosen a laparoscopic removal of the prostate using the robot. I would only stay one night in the hospital and my catheter would have come out in half the time.

If you think you want a nice, mannerly urologist to handle your case, you agree with me. But let me take it a step further. Be sure he is board certified and that he has experience with prostate cancer. Did I get a second opinion? No. Why? My case was not that complicated and I felt confident in Roger's ability.

Schultz

Any responsible doctor will tell you if a second opinion is recommended.

When should you get a second or third opinion?

➤ Any time you are not comfortable with the doctor.

➤ When there is not a clear-cut diagnosis or when you want more information.

➤ When you feel you want a second opinion.

WARNING: You could be in a state of denial if you continue to get numerous opinions.

Communicate, communicate, communicate.

It was difficult and somewhat embarrassing for me to talk about this at first. But talking to others does help. Find at least one person you can be honest with. REMEMBER: Even though it's your prostate, the crisis affects your family, friends, and co-workers. I found that the more I talked about it, the more I helped myself.

Did the doctor know how I felt? You bet, and I had no problem leaning on him. After all, he was not only treating the cancer, he was treating me in other ways.

Learn from other men's experiences.

Schultz: Now let me say one more word here. As a doctor, I have found that a former patient can be a great asset to me. In fact, Alex has spoken with many men since his experience. What he tells them is good, practical medicine:

➢ Get exercise. Stay fit.

➢ Eat sensibly.

➢ Get plenty of rest.

➢ Understand your emotional self. If you feel like you're falling down a well or feel tired and angry, talk it out with someone.

➢ Visit the location for your treatment and know who will be there to help you.

➢ Let your coworkers know what your schedule will be during treatment and how they can help you at work.

➢ Allow friends and neighbors to help you with household chores and other responsibilities. Ask them to keep you in their thoughts and prayers.

This can be a stressful time in your life. Taking care of your total self will help.

I continue to note a great change in men's attitudes about prostate cancer. We are talking about it and want to help other men. This aids the healing process.

Chapter 7

Life After Therapy

Schultz

Believe it or not, you can resume a normal life following treatment for prostate cancer. You may have restricted activities following surgery for a total of four to six weeks. After this time, you can gradually resume just about everything you used to do. The side effects of radiation usually don't last long, so you can expect to feel more normal within several weeks or, more rarely, several months following therapy. Hormonal treatments do not limit your physical activities, but the loss of testosterone (male hormone) can make you feel tired and may cause osteoporosis (loss of calcium from bones).

All of these therapies may have one common side effect—erectile impotence. After surgery or radiation, you may need to wait as long as one or two years to see the return of erectile function. With hormonal therapy, your testosterone levels fall and impotence is permanent. You should not write off your sex life, however, because there are several avenues of treatment for this condition regardless of its cause. Your urologist can show you a vacuum constriction device that mechanically helps you to achieve and hold an erection. There are also pharmacological approaches that use drugs that vasodilate, or open up, the penile blood vessels. The three pills on the market that are available include *Viagra, Levitra* and *Cialis*. Also available is MUSE, a medicated suppository that you place about one inch down the urethra. The pellet melts and causes an erection in ten minutes. Last, there is a drug called *Prostaglandin E-1 (Caverject, Edex)* which you can inject directly into the penis and will cause an erection in ten minutes.

Except for hormonal therapy, you can expect to retain your interest in sex. Orgasm and the rhythmic muscular contractions that accompany the climax can still occur. There is no significant semen with climax because the source of this fluid, the prostate and seminal vesicles, have been removed or irradiated. Although this affects your fertility, it does not pose any risk to your health.

When neither the vacuum pump nor drugs prove satisfactory, we can recommend the placement of a penile prosthesis. The surgery takes one or two hours and can be done with a very minimal hospital stay. The prosthesis is permanent, but you are no more aware of it than you are aware of the shoe on your foot. It can be used any time and any number of times. The greatest advantage of a penile prosthesis is the spontaneity that it offers. There is no prescription and no special preparation involved. Medicare and many insurance carriers often cover the surgical costs.

Fortunately, most men regain urinary control after radical prostatectomy. Some men have very troubling urgency following surgery. This may be due to a bladder made irritable by previous prostatic obstruction. In these instances, we may offer you an anticholinergic pill (e.g., Detrol, Ditropan) to decrease symptoms.

Mild to moderate urinary incontinence can be treated with the *"Male sling"* (*AdVance procedure*). This minimally invasive procedure involves placement of synthetic mesh to elevate the urethra and provide support. It is relatively new, so long term results are not yet known.

On occasion men develop more severe incontinence. In these cases we may recommend the surgical implantation of an *Artificial Urinary Sphincter (AUS)*. Much like the penile implant, an AUS is a simple one hour procedure, often done with minimal hospital stay. A urethral cuff is implanted which is continuously filled with water to close off the urethra. When you need to void, you simply press a scrotally placed pump to force fluid from the urethral cuff to the reservoir. The bladder will drain out of the opened urethra. In three minutes, the urethral cuff automatically refills.

> "My wife, Libbey, tells me that I was tied up in a big knot when I got the news. It was a great deal to think about and I was mostly concerned as to how this could negatively affect my marriage. Libbey worked with me and with time the knot began to unravel. Today my marriage is stronger because of the experience, and the remaining threads of the knot have been woven deeply in the fabric of our lives."
>
> *Alex W. Oliver*

Schultz

I make a big point about follow-up. There is no such thing as a 100% cure rate. Even when we are dealing with locally confined disease, there will be some unfortunate person whose cancer shows up again, either soon after treatment or even years later. Presumably this is due to cancer cells either in the pelvis or in more distant locations. The PSA is the most sensitive marker of recurrent disease. After radical prostatectomy, the PSA should remain undetectable. After successful radiation, the PSA will reach a low level, preferably less than 0.5 ng/ml, and remain in this range forever.

I see my patients several times in the first year following treatment, then less often as time passes without recurrent cancer. At the very least, I see my patients annually. Recurrent cancer is usually first suggested by a rising PSA in a patient without complaints. The PSA may precede the onset of symptoms by many months. Some feel that early and rapid rise in the PSA after treatment means metastatic disease. We treat advancing disease by removing the testicles or giving LHRH agonists (medicines to lower male hormone). A late and slowly rising PSA that occurs several years following treatment may indicate a recurrence in the pelvis. We don't always treat patients whose PSA values rise years after treatment. Often these are patients with no symptoms who will outlive their disease recurrence. You and your doctor would need to decide whether the cancer may hurt you or the treatment may hurt you even more!

Chapter 8

UNEXPECTED REWARDS
Ten Years Later

Alex: Our local newspaper recently reported that an older woman who had been cancer-free for ten years was planning to celebrate by going skydiving. My ten-year celebration was a quiet, uneventful one. It was a time of reflection and appreciation of good health and new experiences that have positively affected my life. The experience of surviving prostate cancer and writing this manual has brought Roger and me together as good friends.

Roger: All men should work toward developing good relationships with their physicians. Trust in your physician, coupled with a clear understanding of the treatment options, plays a significant part in a successful outcome.

I am very grateful to have made friends with Alex and his wife, Libbey. They are truly like family. On the professional side, Alex has taught me to become a better listener. The experience of writing this book and speaking to groups has helped me to communicate more effectively in my personal and professional lives.

Cancer-free vs. Cured
Cancer-free does not mean you are cured! Today you may show no signs of cancer, but recurrences can happen years later. That's why it is important to see the doctor for follow-up examinations.

I want to conclude with an appeal for regular check-ups for men who have been treated for localized prostate cancer. After treatment, your PSA may be zero, but it does not always mean that you have been cured. During scheduled visits, I want to know if my patient is cancer-free and if he has had problems from the therapy itself. The visit includes an examination, a PSA measurement, and often a urinalysis. A rectal mass, a rising PSA, or blood in the urine may suggest active cancer.

Recurrent cancer can be treated, but it may require a different therapy—e.g., radiation therapy if the surgery has failed, cryotherapy for a radiation failure, hormonal or chemotherapy if the cancer is widespread. For the patient with advanced prostate cancer, follow-up visits ensure that hormonal management (shots or testicle removal) keep the cancer in check. The office visit allows us to discuss side effects of hormonal deprivation or chemotherapy.

You should see the doctor twice a year for the first five years and then plan to schedule an annual examination for the rest of your life. The urologist should send your reports to your internist or to your primary care physician.

If you move to another location, please take a copy of your medical records. Your next medical team needs to know important details such as your pre-treatment exam, PSA, and biopsy reports. Surgical records and a surgical pathology report, or a summary letter from the radiation or medical oncologist, are enormously helpful. Finally, you should bring a listing of your PSA levels since you were treated. There are pages in the back of this manual for recording these reports.

Alex: Roger and I have spent time speaking to support groups and local clubs about prostate cancer and health advocacy. We have

It helps to know that your hospital is accredited as a cancer center of excellence. Many hospitals have received accreditation from the American Cancer Society. These hospitals keep careful records of all patients treated with cancer. They survey their medical staff and send outcomes data to a central registry. This activity adds one additional layer of oversight that may give you greater confidence in your selection of a facility for your treatment.

spoken to a growing number of younger men, often in their forties, who have been diagnosed with prostate cancer. Thanks to screening and early detection, their cancers are usually caught early enough to be effectively treated.

Roger: Men have become more open and honest about their medical concerns, but there are still too many men who do not go to the doctor until there are symptoms, such as difficulty urinating or blood in the urine. By the time these symptoms occur the cancer is usually much larger and more difficult to treat. More men are aware of the importance of exercise and good nutrition. It makes sense for men beyond age fifty to get an annual physical, even if they are feeling well.

Alex: Let's get back to the red dot and yellow square on the cover. In a previous chapter, we discussed the meaning of the graphic element. For me, the dot that represents prostate cancer has not gone. Today, it is a smaller dot that represents one of the many significant experiences in my life. On the yellow square that represents my life, there are also red dots for education, marriage, and other important life accomplishments. I have recently added other red dots: one for writing this book and another for my friendship with Roger and his family. These new dots represent the unexpected rewards of surviving prostate cancer.

We hope that our book will be a help to many men and their loved ones and that upon recovery, you, too, will value the unexpected rewards by helping others.

Glossary

Antiandrogens—Oral drugs (Eulexin, Casodex, Nilandron) that block the effects of testosterone. Often used together with either orchiectomies or LHRH agonists in an effort to improve survival.

Brachytherapy (Interstitial radiation)—The placement of radioactive seeds into the substance of the prostate to destroy cancer cells. The seeds are permanently implanted and become inert after many months.

Complete Androgen Blockade—The combination of orchiectomies and antiandrogens, or LHRH agonists and antiandrogens. This will block the production and/or effects of the testosterone produced by the testicles and adrenal glands. It is used in advanced cancer to produce a *remission*.

Cryoablative Surgery—An out-patient procedure during which solid needles are placed into the prostate in order to freeze the entire gland. After freezing and thawing the needles, they are removed. Also known as cryotherapy.

Digital Rectal Examination—The placement of a finger in the rectum to feel the prostate for its size and shape. Lumps (nodules) are considered unusual and could be cancer.

External beam irradiation—Treatment of prostate cancer by aiming a linear accelerator at the cancer to destroy it. Treatments are given during brief daily visits over an eight week period.

Gleason Score—A system for determining the prognosis. The pathologist views the cancer under the microscope to determine the two most common grades (see Grade). These numbers are added together to give the Gleason score. This can range from 2 (1+1) to 10 (5+5). Higher Gleason scores suggest a worse prognosis.

Grade—A means of deciding the speed of growth of a cancer by looking at the cancer cells under the microscope. Prostate cancer is graded from 1-5. The higher the grade, the more aggressive the tumor.

Hormonal deprivation—Prostate cancer often shrinks away when it is deprived of the hormone, testosterone. Testosterone can be reduced by removing the testicles or giving LHRH agonists that lower the body's testosterone levels.

Levaquin—A quinolone antibiotic used to treat prostatitis. It is also used to prevent a bacterial urinary infection following biopsy of the prostate.

LHRH Agonists—Drugs (*Vantas, Zoladex, Eligard, Trelstar and Lupron*) that lower the body's testosterone (male hormone) level.

Margins—The edges of a prostate that have been removed. A pathologist examines these areas closely to be certain that all of the cancer was removed.

Metastatic disease—The condition in which cancer has spread beyond the organ from which it originated. When prostate cancer is found in an organ other than the prostate, it is termed a "metastasis."

Oncologist—A doctor who specializes in the medical treatment of cancers. An oncologist can be involved in the non-surgical treatment of advanced prostate cancer.

Orchiectomies—The surgical removal of the testicles. This is done to reduce blood testosterone levels and put the prostate cancer in remission.

Palliation—Refers to efforts to control the tumor and the symptoms it may produce. Palliation does not mean "cure." Generally, the term is used with patients who have advanced cancer.

Pathologist—A doctor who specializes in the diagnosis of disease by the examination of human tissue that has been removed. These tissues are examined visually and often examined under a microscope.

Percent Free–PSA—A blood test that measures how much PSA is free versus how much is bound to other blood proteins. This may help determine if cancer is present in situations when the regular PSA test is borderline high or rising.

Prostate Specific Antigen—A blood test of an enzyme made almost exclusively by the prostate. The test can be used to screen for prostate cancer. It is especially useful to monitor the results of treatment.

Radiation oncologist—A doctor who specializes in the treatment of cancer using radiation to kill the tumor cells.

Radical prostatectomy—The surgical removal of the entire prostate gland and paired seminal vesicles.

Recurrence—Condition in which the tumor shows up again in the body despite earlier treatment.

Remission—Condition in which the tumor may become invisible, dormant, inactive. Often symptoms may disappear. This can occur commonly in patients who choose hormonal deprivation for advanced cancer. Remissions do not mean "cure." The cancer will probably grow and cause symptoms again later.

Seminal vesicles—Paired organs at the bladder base that empty seminal fluid into the ejaculatory duct when a man reaches his climax. They are usually removed during a radical prostatectomy.

Stage—Describes whether the cancer is locally confined to the prostate or has spread beyond the capsule of the prostate to lymph nodes, bones, liver, lung, or other organs.

Urologist—A doctor who specializes in diseases of the urinary system, particularly those of the kidney, bladder, prostate, and testicles.

Vantas—A soft, plastic, one inch long tube filled with a LHRH agonist (medication) that lowers male hormone levels. It is placed under the skin of the upper arm and dispenses the drug over a year's time. It must be removed in the urologist's office after twelve months and may be replaced with a new implant.

Zolendronic acid (Zometa)—An intravenous drug that has been approved for patients who have prostate cancer in the bones (metastatic disease). It is not chemotherapy. It is given monthly in the doctor's office to reduce the complications of bone fracture, the need for radiation to treat bone pain, and the need for bone surgery to an already weakened bone.

Patient Checklist

Important questions to ask your doctor that will help you choose a course of action.

➤ What is the serum PSA level
    (prostate specific antigen blood test)?

➤ Are you confident in the biopsy diagnosis of prostate cancer? Was there any hesitation by the pathologist to call it cancer? (If so, consider getting the microscope slides reviewed by a second pathologist.)

➤ Regarding the prostate biopsy:
    ➤ What is the Gleason grade and score?
    ➤ How many samples (tissue cores) showed cancer present?

➤ What is the stage of my disease? Has it spread?

➤ Do we want to treat this disease at all, or simply watch it?

➤ If we treat it, what is the treatment that can offer a cure?

➤ Is the disease beyond cure?

➤ How can I prepare mentally, emotionally and spiritually for treatment and healing?

Questions

You Want to Ask the Doctor Throughout Your Treatment

Comments

Your Doctor Makes to You Throughout Treatment

Diagnostic Record

DATE	TYPE OF TEST	RESULT

Notes

About the Authors

Roger E. Schultz, M.D., FACS

Roger E. Schultz, M.D., FACS, is a urologist in private practice with Hampton Roads Urology (a division of Riverside Medical Group) in Williamsburg, Virginia. He is a native of New Jersey and a graduate of Tulane University. He received his medical degree from Mount Sinai School of Medicine in New York and completed his residency at the Hospital of the University of Pennsylvania in Philadelphia. Before entering private practice, he served as staff urologist at the Naval Hospital in Portsmouth, Virginia.

Dr. Schultz has been in private practice since 1989. He is a Fellow of the American College of Surgeons. He served as Chief of Staff at Williamsburg Community Hospital and is a former President of the Tidewater and the Virginia Urological Societies. He has also been President of the Mid-Atlantic Section of the American Urology Association. He continues to serve on national committees of the American Urological Association.

Dr. Schultz lives in Williamsburg with his wife Beth Scharlop, MD. They have two children, Alison and Sam. Dr. Schultz is a clarinetist with the Bagels and Fraylox Klezmer Band.

Alex W. Oliver

Alex W. Oliver has more than twenty years of executive experience with businesses and non-profit organizations, including managing the Chesapeake Division of the Hampton Roads Chamber of Commerce, the Hampton Roads Utility Contractors Association and the Hermitage Foundation Museum. He recently began a consultant practice and works with non-profit organizations and businesses in the Williamsburg area on both long and short term management projects. Some of his recent and current clients include BP America, Sentara Williamsburg Regional Medical Center and Port Warwick Merchants Association. He and his wife Libbey reside in Williamsburg with their two cats, Dandy and Duchess.

CPSIA information can be obtained at www.ICGtesting.com
Printed in the USA
LVOW13s0224141113

361248LV00007B/186/P